Department of Veterans Affairs
Health Services Research & Development Service | Evidence-based Synthesis Program

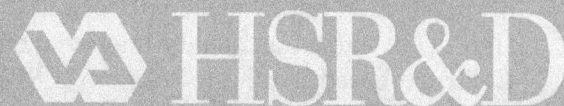

Self-Monitoring of Blood Glucose in Patients with Type 2 Diabetes Mellitus: Meta Analysis of Effectiveness

September 2007

Prepared for:

Department of Veterans Affairs
Veterans Health Administration
Health Services Research & Development Service
Washington, DC 20420

Prepared by:

Greater Los Angeles Veterans Affairs Healthcare System/Southern California/RAND Evidence-based Practice Center
Los Angeles, CA

Investigators:

Paul Shekelle, MD, PhD
Director

Brett Munjas, BA
Project Manager/Literature Database Manager

Maria Romanova, MD
Ali Towfigh, MD
Physician Reviewers

Jane Weinreb, MD
Content Expert

Annie Zhou, MS
Marika Suttorp, MS
Statisticians

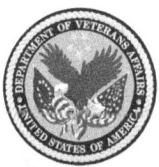

PREFACE

VA's Health Services Research and Development Service (HSR&D) works to improve the cost, quality, and outcomes of health care for our nation's veterans. Collaborating with VA leaders, managers, and policy makers, HSR&D focuses on important health care topics that are likely to have significant impact on quality improvement efforts. One significant collaborative effort is HSR&D's Evidence-based Synthesis Program (ESP). Through this program, HSR&D provides timely and accurate evidence syntheses on targeted health care topics. These products will be disseminated broadly throughout VA and will: inform VA clinical policy, develop clinical practice guidelines, set directions for future research to address gaps in knowledge, identify the evidence to support VA performance measures, and rationalize drug formulary decisions.

HSR&D provided funding for the two Evidence Based Practice Centers (EPCs) supported by the Agency for Healthcare Research and Quality (AHRQ) that also had an active and publicly acknowledged VA affiliation—Southern California EPC and Portland, OR EPC—so they could develop evidence syntheses on requested topics for dissemination to VA policymakers. A planning committee with representation from HSR&D, Patient Care Services, Office of Quality and Performance, and the VISN Clinical Management Officers, has been established to identify priority topics and to insure the quality of final reports.

Comments on this evidence report are welcome and can be sent to Susan Schiffner, ESP Program Manager, at Susan.Schiffner@va.gov.

EXECUTIVE SUMMARY

BACKGROUND

Diabetes is a prevalent and costly disease in Veterans. Control of blood glucose is an important VA objective. Self-monitoring of blood glucose (SMBG) is advocated as a method to better achieve control.

The Key Questions were:

>   Key Question 1. Is regular SMBG effective in achieving target A1c levels for patients with type 2 diabetes?

>   Key Question 2. Is regular SMBG effective in maintaining target A1c levels for patients with type 2 diabetes?

>   Key Question 3. Does regular SMBG reduce the frequency of hypoglycemia in patients with type 2 diabetes?

>   Key Question 4. Is there evidence that different frequencies of testing result in differences in improvements in A1c?

METHODS

We searched PubMed from 2004-2006 using standard search terms. We performed an update search in July 2007. Titles, abstracts, and articles were reviewed in duplicate by physicians trained in the critical analysis of literature. Data were extracted by quantitative analysts. Pooled analyses were performed for trials with A1c outcomes at six months and 12 months or greater of follow-up. All other data were narratively summarized.

RESULTS

We screened 52 titles, 14 were rejected, and we performed a more detailed review on 38 articles. From this, we identified 14 randomized controlled trials (RCTs) that measured the effect of SMBG compared to a group not receiving SMBG and monitored A1c levels with at least three months of follow-up. Four trials were excluded; one because it presented duplicate data and three because they evaluated SMBG in both the control and intervention groups, leaving 10 trials contributing to the efficacy analysis. We identified five observational studies assessing effectiveness in diabetic Veterans.

KEY QUESTION #1: Is regular SMBG effective in achieving target A1c levels for patients with type 2 diabetes?

STUDIES OF EFFICACY
Achieving Target A1c Levels
There is little evidence to draw a conclusion about the effect of SMBG at achieving target A1c levels. We judged the strength of this evidence as very low. [GRADE: Very Low = Any estimate of effect is very uncertain.]

Improving Glycemic Control

We found that adding SMBG along with education, counseling, (and some times other components) results in a statistically significant decrease in A1c level of an absolute 0.21% at six months. Results at three months and one year are more variable, although there is a suggestion that this benefit may continue out to at least one year.

We judged the strength of evidence for this outcome as moderate, because individual trials did not in general report significant results and interventions were heterogeneous. [GRADE: Moderate= Further research is likely to have an important impact on our confidence in the estimate of effect and may change the estimate.]

STUDIES OF EFFECTIVENESS IN VETERANS

Five observational studies of SMBG effectiveness in Veteran populations did not report statistically significant improvements in glycemic control. [GRADE: Very Low = Any estimate of effect is very uncertain.]

KEY QUESTION #2: Is regular SMBG effective in maintaining target A1c levels for patients with type 2 diabetes?

We did not identify any trials that directly assessed this question. Therefore, we draw no conclusion and the strength of evidence is very low. [GRADE: Very Low = Any estimate of effect is very uncertain.]

KEY QUESTION #3: Does regular SMBG reduce the frequency of hypoglycemia in patients with type 2 diabetes?

The limited evidence available indicates that SMBG increases the frequency of recognized hypoglycemia. This is due to an increase in asymptomatic low blood sugar readings, and also an increase in mild-to-moderate symptomatic episodes. There is scant evidence about the effect of SMBG on more clinically significant hypoglycemia. We judge the strength of evidence for SMBG increasing asymptomatic and mildly symptomatic hypoglycemia as moderate. [Moderate = Further research is likely to have an important impact on our confidence in the estimate of effect and may change the estimate.]

KEY QUESTION #4: Is there evidence that different frequencies of testing result in differences in improvements in A1c?

We used meta-regression to assess the effect of the reported frequency of SMBG use in the RCTs (measures as times/week) on differences in A1c level compared to control. No association was found (p=0.99). Therefore we draw no conclusion about the effect of frequency of SMBG monitoring on A1c values, and judge the strength of the evidence to be very low. [GRADE: Very Low = Any estimate of effect is very uncertain.]

TABLE OF CONTENTS

In-Text Figure and Tables

INTRODUCTION

Background

According to the World Health Organization, at least 180 million people worldwide suffer from diabetes. [1] Though prevalent throughout the world, diabetes is more common (especially type 2) in more developed countries like the United States. The National Diabetes Information Clearinghouse estimates that diabetes costs $132 billion in the United States alone every year. [2] Given these estimates along with the projection that the worldwide incidence of diabetes will double in the next 20 years, [1] intensified research into better management of this chronic disease is paramount.

Tighter control of blood glucose is advocated as a means to reduce microvascular and macrovascular complications. [3] VA has performance measures assessing the proportion of patients meeting certain A1c goals, currently 7% and 9%. Theoretically, self-monitoring of blood glucose (SMBG) can improve compliance with recommendations on diet and exercise and medication regimens. The American Diabetes Association has recommended that the optimal frequency of SMBG for patients with type 2 diabetes should be adequate to facilitate reaching glucose goals. This hypothesis is based on the expectation that life style changes are facilitated by SMBG. Under these conditions, we should expect an improvement of glycemic control SMBG may decrease patient management costs, and because of the high prevalence of type 2 diabetes, efforts to establish the efficacy of SMBG in type 2 diabetes mellitus are of greater relevance. Methods to achieve improved glycemic control, and therefore a higher proportion of patients meeting target A1c levels, include diet, exercise, and medication. However, evidence supporting the use of SMBG for diabetics not requiring insulin is not as clear.

The purpose of this review is to analyze the literature to answer four key questions given to us by VA: 1) Is regular self-monitoring of blood glucose effective in achieving target A1c levels for patients with type 2 diabetes?; 2) Is regular self-monitoring of blood glucose effective in maintaining target A1c levels for patients with type 2 diabetes?; 3) Does regular self-monitoring of blood glucose reduce the frequency of hypoglycemia in patients with type 2 diabetes?; 4) Is there evidence that different frequencies of testing result in differences in improvements in A1c?

METHODS

Topic Development

This project was nominated by Dr. Chester B. Good, from the VA Pharmacy service for the Evidence Synthesis Project. Key questions were discussed and finalized during a conference call that included the Steering Committee of the Evidence Synthesis Project and the VA Greater Los Angeles project site director. The final key questions are:

1. Is regular SMBG effective in achieving target A1c levels for patients with type 2 diabetes?

2. Is regular SMBG effective in maintaining target A1c levels for patients with type 2 diabetes?

3. Does regular SMBG reduce the frequency of hypoglycemia in patients with type 2 diabetes?

4. Is there evidence that different frequencies of testing result in differences in improvements in A1c?

Search Strategy

This topic has been the subject of several previous reviews.

Faas et al. (1997) [4] This review covered the years 1976-1996 and identified 11 studies from two Medline searches that met the inclusion criteria. Studies were excluded if they were not RCTs and if the patients were exclusively using insulin.

Coster et al. (2000) [5] This review covered the years 1990-1999 and originally identified 18 possibly relevant studies. Non-randomized studies were excluded. The review included eight randomized controlled trials. Two additional randomized trials were excluded; one because it used fructosamine as an outcome and the other because it used cluster randomization.

Welschen et al. (2005) [6] This review covered the years 1966 to 2004. A total of 36 articles were retrieved for further review of which five trials were included in the review. A total of six articles, one in press during the time of the initial search, were examined. Included trials looked at the effectiveness of SMBG compared with usual care in patients with type 2 diabetes who were not using insulin at the start of the trial and studies comparing SMBG and urine glucose monitoring.

Balk et al. (2006, draft report for AHRQ) [7] At the time we received this draft report by the Tufts-NEMC EPC it had only been distributed for the purpose of peer review and discussion at the Medicare Coverage Advisory committee meeting and had not yet been disseminated by the Agency for Healthcare Research and Quality. This review, dated August 16, 2006, identified five RCTs that evaluated SMBG with A1c as the outcome. Reasons for exclusion from this review were wrong population (type 1 diabetes), sample size too small (for inclusion n≥100 in the intervention arm), follow-up time too short (for non-clinical outcomes follow-up time had to be greater than or equal to three months), intervention or outcome not of interest, design (cross-sectional or retrospective), or the trial contained no primary data or duplicate data.

Jansen (2006) [8] This review covered the years 1966-2005. The review included studies that evaluated SMBG versus no self-monitoring, SMBG versus self-monitoring of urine glucose and SMBG with regular feedback versus monitoring without feedback. The review identified 27 studies that underwent quality assessment, from which 14 trials were excluded due to the outcome they assessed, type of diabetes included or the intervention was not clearly described.

The Balk et al. [7] review was not available to us at the start of this project. We judged the search strategy and inclusion/exclusion criteria of the review by Welschen et al. [6] to be comprehensive and therefore acceptable as the basis for our own review. We updated this search by searching PubMed from the end date of the prior search to October, 2006 and performed an update search in July 2007.

The search strategy is listed below:

DATABASE SEARCHED & TIME PERIOD COVERED:
PUBMED – 2004-2006

LIMITERS:

SEARCH STRATEGY:
Randomized Controlled Trail AND
Diabetes Mellitus, Type 2 AND
Blood Glucose self-monitoring

NUMBER OF ITEMS RETRIEVED: 23

In addition to our PubMed search and screening references from prior reviews, we also performed reference mining of retrieved articles.

Study Selection

Two trained researchers reviewed the list of titles and selected articles for further review. The team of researchers consisted of two general internists, one with a special interest in diabetes. Each article retrieved was reviewed with a brief screening form (see Appendix A) that collected data on efficacy or effectiveness of SMBG alone or as part of a multi-component intervention, A1c and hypoglycemia reported as outcomes, the report of frequency of SMBG, duration of follow-up, study design, and whether or not the subjects in the study were Veterans. To be included in our evidence report, a study had to measure the efficacy or effectiveness of SMBG alone or as part of a multi-component intervention and have a follow up duration greater than or equal to 12 weeks (chosen because of the use of A1c as the outcome measure). Eligible study designs for efficacy included controlled clinical trials, RCTs, and systematic reviews/meta-analyses. Observational studies, case reports, non-systematic reviews, letters to the editor and other similar contributions were excluded as evidence of efficacy. To assess effectiveness, we required that studies assess SMBG in a Veteran population and VA healthcare delivery setting. RCTs and observational studies were eligible.

Data Abstraction

Data were independently abstracted by two general internists trained in critical reading of the literature, with consensus resolution. The following data were abstracted from included trials: design; randomization and appropriateness; blinding and appropriateness; withdrawals and dropouts described; sample size enrolled and followed-up; characteristics of the population including percent women and race; mean, median, and range of age; mean, median and range of BMI; mean, median and range of duration of diabetes; reported co-morbidities; sample size and intervention/exposure data for each arm of the study (intervention/exposure data included components of the intervention, total number of visits, frequency of SMBG, number of days per week monitored, duration of treatment, co-therapies); outcomes measured; intervals in which the outcomes were measured; adverse events. Data abstraction forms are provided in Appendix A. The mean A1c level and standard deviation was collected by treatment arm for each reported follow-up point. For trials that reported a mean outcome but no standard deviation, we estimated the standard deviation by taking the unweighted mean standard deviation across all other trials that reported standard deviations for the A1c level. [9]

Quality assessment

To assess internal validity of diagnostic studies, we used the Delphi criteria[10] (see Appendix A). We abstracted data on treatment allocation; was the method of randomization performed and was the treatment allocation concealed; were the groups similar at baseline regarding the most important prognostic indicators; were the eligibility criteria specified; was the outcome assessor blinded; was the care provider blinded; was the patient blinded; were point estimates and measures of variability presented for the primary outcome measures; did the analysis include an intention-to-treat analysis. Our own work [11] supports using a threshold of four for distinguishing "high" versus "low" quality studies.

Data Synthesis

Of the articles that were determined to be clinically eligible, duration of follow-up and frequency of SMBG were reviewed across studies to see if they were comparable.

Since the outcome of interest was the same across all trials, a mean difference was calculated for each time point that reported statistical data. The mean difference is the difference between the follow-up mean A1c level for the SMBG group and the follow-up mean A1c level for the control group. A negative mean difference indicates that the SMBG group has a lower mean A1c score than the control group. For our main analysis, we did not control for the baseline mean A1c for each group (a difference of differences estimate) since there is evidence that this approach is susceptible to bias. [12] We presented results controlling for the baseline as a sensitivity analysis.

A pooled estimate was calculated by follow-up time, in the following categories: 3- 6months, 6-11 months, and 12 months or greater. The pooled estimate was calculated using the DerSimonian & Laird[13] random effects model. In addition, we calculated a pooled estimate stratified by high and low quality trials.

Meta-regressions[14] were performed to individually examine the effect of treatment frequency, quality score, and the baseline A1c mean on the mean difference. For trials with more than one follow-up time, the long term estimates were used.

Test of heterogeneity were performed using Cochran's Q[15] and the I^2 statistic. [16] A significant Q statistic or I^2 values close to 100% represent very high degrees of heterogeneity. Publication bias was examined using the Begg rank correlation and Egger regression asymmetry test. All analyses were conducted in Stata 9.2. [17]

Rating the body of evidence

We assessed the overall quality of evidence for outcomes using a method developed by the Grade Working Group, which classified the grade of evidence across outcomes according to the following criteria: [18]

- o **High** = Further research is very unlikely to change our confidence on the estimate of effect.
- o **Moderate** = Further research is likely to have an important impact on our confidence in the estimate of effect and may change the estimate.
- o **Low** = Further research is very likely to have an important impact on our confidence in the estimate of effect and is likely to change the estimate.
- o **Very Low** = Any estimate of effect is very uncertain.

GRADE also suggests using the following scheme for assigning the "grade" or strength of evidence:

Criteria for assigning grade of evidence
Type of evidence Randomized trial = high Observational study = low Any other evidence = very low
Decrease grade if: • Serious (-1) or very serious (-2) limitation to study quality • Important inconsistency (-1) • Some (-1) or major (-2) uncertainty about directness • Imprecise or sparse data (-1) • High probability of reporting bias (-1)
Increase grade if: • Strong evidence of association-significant relative risk of > 2 (< 0.5) based on consistent evidence from two or more observational studies, with no plausible confounders (+1) • Very strong evidence of association-significant relative risk of > 5 (< 0.2) based on direct evidence with no major threats to validity (+2) • Evidence of a dose response gradient (+1) • All plausible confounders would have reduced the effect (+1)

For this report, we used both this explicit scoring scheme and the global implicit judgment about "confidence" in the result. Where the two disagreed, we went with the lower of the two classifications.

Peer Review

A draft version of this report was sent to three peer reviewers. Their comments and our responses are presented in Appendix B.

RESULTS

Literature Flow

In total, we examined 52 titles. Seventeen articles were identified from prior systematic reviews. The electronic update search identified 23 articles. An additional 11 articles were identified through reference mining. One was identified by a content expert.

Of the titles identified through our electronic literature search, 14 were rejected as not relevant to the project. This left 38 from all sources. Ten articles were excluded at abstract review. In January 2006 we received the Balk and colleagues draft report of a review of SMBG in type 2 diabetes.[7]

We performed an update search in July of 2007 that resulted in two additional articles, one of which was excluded since it did not test SMBG. In total we reviewed 30 articles.

We compared trials identified for our review with those identified in the three recent systematic reviews (Table 1). Our review included 10 trials, compared to six in the review by Welschen and colleagues,[6] seven in the review by Balk and colleagues,[7] and 13 in the review by Jansen.[8] Jansen included studies of self-monitoring of urine glucose that we did not, and we included studies rejected by Balk and/or by Welschen for a variety of reasons, detailed in Table 1.

Initial screening of the articles resulted in 14 RCTs that measured the effect of SMBG compared to a group not receiving SMBG and monitored A1c levels with at least three months of follow-up. Four were excluded; one because the trial presented duplicate data, the other three because the trials compared a control group of SMBG to an intervention group of SMBG plus other components. (Figure 1) We identified five observational studies that assessed the effectiveness of SMBG in diabetic Veterans.

Description of the Efficacy Evidence

The 10 RCTs ranged in size from 29 to 988 subjects. All patients had type 2 diabetes, the mean duration of which was three to 13 years. All trials but one included only patients treated without insulin, the one exception being a trial from Bangladesh that included patients on oral hypoglycemic agents or insulin and not specifying how many of each type. The average age of patients was between 50 and 66. Almost all trials included counseling/education with SMBG in the intervention group, but other components of the intervention were varied (Table 2).
All trials measured A1c as an outcome; five trials assessed this at six months, three trials assessed this at three months, and five trials assessed this at one year or more. The quality of trials varied; most trials scored positively on less then half of the criteria on the Delphi list.[10] Details of each trial are presented in the Evidence Table (Appendix C). We now present a brief synopsis of each trial.

Table 1. Comparison of RCTs we included in our review with those included in three recent systematic reviews.

	Welschen (2005)[6]	Balk (2006)[7]	Jansen (2006)[8]	Our Review	Comments
Wing RR, Epstein LH, Nowalk MP et al. Does self-monitoring of blood glucose levels improve dietary compliance for obese patients with type II diabetes? Am J Med. 1986 Nove; 81(5):830-6. [19]			X	X	
Fontbonne A, Billault B, Acosta M et al. Is glucose self-monitoring beneficial in non-insulin-treated diabetic patients? Results of a randomized comparative trial. *Diabete Metab.* 1989 Sept-1989 Oct 31; 15(5):255-60. [20]	X	X	X	X	
Estey AL, Tan MH, Mann K. Follow-up intervention: its effect on compliance behavior to a diabetes regimen. *Diabetes Educ.* 1990 Jul-1990 Aug 31; 16(4):291-5. [21]			X		Excluded in our review because it evaluated SMBG vs. SMBG plus other components.
Allen BT, DeLong ER, Feussner JR. Impact of glucose self-monitoring on non-insulin-treated patients with type II diabetes mellitus: Randomized controlled trial comparing blood and urine testing. *Diabetes Care.* 1990 Oct; 13(10):1044-50. [22]	X		X		Excluded in our review due to the comparison of SMBG to self-monitoring of urine glucose (SMUG).
Rutten G, van Eijk J, de Noebl E, et al. Feasibility and effects of a diabetes type II protocol with blood glucose self-monitoring in general practice. *Fam Pract.* 1990 Dec; 7(4):273-8. [23]		X	X	X	
Muchmore DB, Springer J, Miller M. Self-monitoring of blood glucose in overweight type 2 diabetic patients. *Acta Diabetol.* 1994 Dec; 31(4):215-09 [24]	X		X	X	
Jaber LA, Halapy H, Fernet M, et al. Evaluation of a pharmaceutical care model on diabetes management. *Ann Pharmacother.* 1996 Mar; 30(2):238-43. [25]			X	X	
Miles P. Everett J, Murphy J et al. Comparison of blood or urine testing by patients with newly diagnosed non-insulin dependent diabetes: patient survey after randomized crossover trial. *BMJ.* 1997 Aug 9; 315(7104):348-9. [26]		X	X		Excluded in our study because it tested SMBG versus self-monitoring of urine glucose.
Kibriya, MG, Ali L, Banik NG, et al. Home monitoring of blood glucose (HMBG) in Type-2 diabetes mellitus in a developing country. *Diabetes Res Clin Pract.* 1999 Dec; 46(3):253-7. [27]		X		X	
Brown SA, Garcia AA, Kouzekanani K at al. Culturally competent diabetes self-management education for Mexican Americans: the Starr County boarder health initiative. *Diabetes Care.* 2002 Feb; 25(2):259-68. [28]			X		Excluded as the primary focus of the study was delivering culturally competent diabetes self management education.
Schwedes U, Siebolds M, Mertes G. Meal-related structured self-monitoring of blood glucose: effect on diabetes control in non-insulin-treated type 2 diabetic patients. *Diabetes Care.* 2002 Nov; 25(11):1928-32. [29]	X	X	X	X	
Guerci B, Drouin P, Grange V, et al. Self-monitoring of blood glucose significantly improves metabolic control in patients with type 2 diabetes mellitus: the Auto-Surveillance Intervention Active (ASIA) study. *Diabetes Metab.* 2003 Dec; 29(6):587-94. [30]	X	X	X	X	
Kwon HS, Cho JH, Him HS et al. Establishment of blood glucose monitoring system using the internet. *Diabetes Care.* 2004 Feb; 27(2):478-83. [31]			X		Excluded because control group also used SMBG.
Davidson MB, Castellanos M, Kain D et al. The effect of self-monitoring of blood glucose concentrations on glycated hemoglobin levels in diabetic patients not taking insulin: a blinded, randomized trail. *Am J Med.* 2005 Apr; 118(4):422-5. [32]	X	X	X	X	
Farmer A, Wade A, Goyder E, et al. Impact of self monitoring of blood glucose in the management of patients with non-insulin treated diabetes: open parallel group randomized trial. *BMJ.* 2007 [33]				X	

Figure 1. Self-monitoring of Blood Glucose Literature Flow

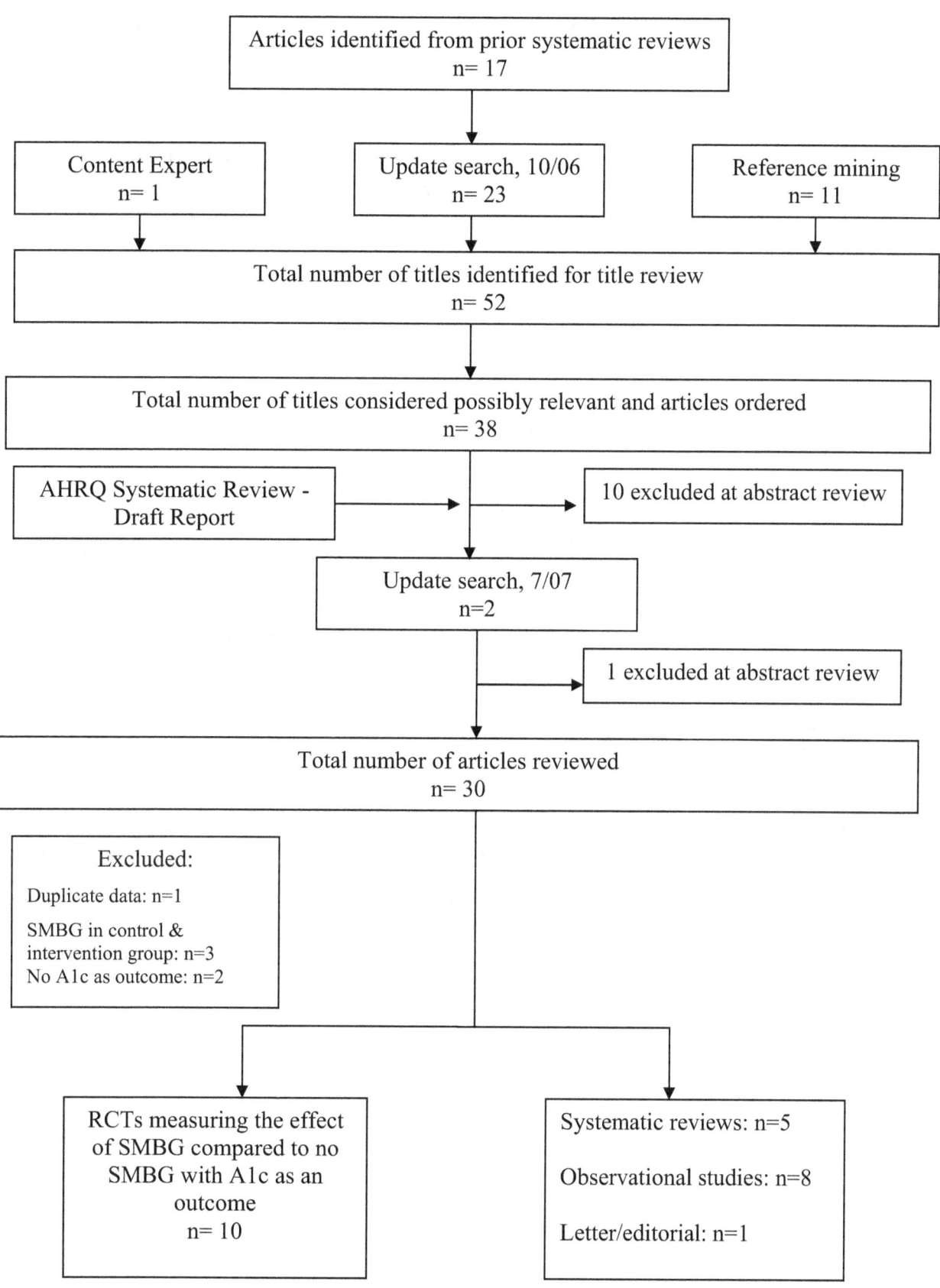

Wing RR et al. (1986) [19] This study assessed the usefulness of SMBG in improvement of dietary compliance for obese patients with type 2 diabetes. Authors from the University of Pittsburgh School of Medicine enrolled 50 patients (mean weight 98 kg, 78% women) with adult-onset diabetes who were treated with oral hypoglycemic agents and insulin. All patients received weekly behavioral weight control counseling for the first three months, then monthly for six months, and twice more until week 62. Monetary stimulation was used. The intervention group was asked to monitor blood glucose on average 5.4 times a week to provide feedback of dietary modifications. Patients' compliance with the diet and SMBG were monitored. Medication adjustments were made in similar mode in both groups according to study protocol. Five patients were excluded from the analyses with reasons explained by the authors. By week 12 there was a slight improvement of glycemic control in both groups (A1c values: SMBG group: 10.19% to 9.68%, control group: 10.86% to 10%). No statistically significant difference between groups was observed in glycosylated hemoglobin measurements by the one-year follow up. Both groups lost a significant amount of weight (6.1 kg). Patients with a high level of compliance to either SMBG or weight loss lost twice the amount of weight compared to poorly compliant patients. A large and not significantly different number of patients in both groups had their medications or insulin dose decreased during the study.

Table 2. Components of each arm of the 10 RCTs.

	Study Arm	SMBG	Counseling/ Education	Dietician	Exercise	Carbohydrate Counting	Financial Incentive (weight)	Financial Incentive (SMBG)	Patient Control
Wing RR et al., 1986[19]	Control		X				X	X	
	Intervention	X	X				X	X	
Fontebonne A et al., 1989[20]	Control		X						
	Intervention	X	X						
Rutten G et al., 1990[23]	Control		X						
	Intervention	X							
Muchmore DB et al., 1994[24]	Control		X	X					
	Intervention	X	X	X		X			
Jaber LA et al., 1996[25]	Control								
	Intervention	X	X		X				
Kibriya MG et al., 1999[27]	Control		X						
	Intervention	X	X						
Schwedes U et al., 2002[29]	Control		X						
	Intervention	X	X						
Guerci B et al. 2003[30]	Control		X						
	Intervention	X	X						
Davidson MB et al., 2005[32]	Control		X	X					
	Intervention	X	X	X					
Farmer A et al. 2007[33]	Control								
	Intervention1	X							
	Intervention2	X							X

Fontbonne A et al. (1989) [20] This is a French study of 208 non-insulin treated patients with long-term and poorly controlled diabetes (mean duration=13 years, mean A1c=8.3%). Patients were randomized into three groups (SMBG, urinary glucose monitoring and control), and seen by their respective physicians every two months with either A1c results or SMBG measurements. At each visit medication and/or dietary modification was allowed. Forty-four patients were lost to follow-up. A1c values at the end of six months were not significantly different between the three groups. However, the degree of compliance to SMBG appeared to relate to outcome; the more blood strips used, the larger the decrease in A1c values.

Rutten G et al. (1990) [23] This study from the Netherlands looked at the feasibility and effect of a diabetes type 2 protocol with SMBG in general practice. One hundred forty-nine patients (66 in intervention and 83 in control groups) from eight practices were studied over 12 months. Ten patients were excluded from each group with reasons explained for all. Some patients in the treatment group tested their fasting glucose and reported it on a monthly basis. In case of elevated readings, they were referred to a study doctor, where the protocol was followed and medications were possibly changed. The protocol included weight reduction counseling and medication changes with up to two oral hypoglycemic agents used. Other patients from the treatment group did not check their blood glucose, but had it measured during quarter-annual visits with a doctor. At the end of the study, the treatment group decreased A1c values from 9.7% to 9.2%, whereas the control group increased from 8.9% to 9.4%.

Muchmore DB et al. (1994) [24] This study tested the hypothesis that combined use of SMBG and dietary carbohydrate counting is beneficial in managing type 2 diabetes. The Scripps Clinic enrolled 29 overweight patients (BMI=34, 61% women) with diet or treated with oral hypoglycemics diabetes. Six were excluded for reasons not described. Patients participated in a 28-week behavioral weight loss program, with emphasis on glycemic response to carbohydrate intake and exercise. Medication adjustment was not included in the study protocol, but it was done for a similar amount of patients in both groups by their own physicians. Although A1c improved more in the intervention group than in the control group (a decrease of 1.54% vs. 0.84% absolute), the difference was not statistically significant. Quality-of-life measures were similar in both groups. Weight loss was equivalent (~6 kg) in both groups by week 44.

Jaber LA et al. (1996) [25] This study was performed in a university-affiliated internal medicine outpatient clinic. It enrolled 45 obese African-American patients with non-insulin dependent diabetes mellitus (NIDDM). All patients were treated with sulfonylurea agents. The mean age of the patients was 62, 70% were women, the mean BMI was 33, and mean duration of diabetes was six years. During four months of follow-up, the intervention group received diabetic education, medication counseling, instructions on dietary regulation, exercise, and SMBG, as well as evaluation and adjustment of their hypoglycemic regimen by the pharmacist. Patients were instructed to monitor blood glucose eight times a week. The control group was followed by their physicians. Six patients withdrew or dropped out from the study with reasons explained by the authors. The intervention group patients had on average 2.2 changes in drug therapy, with an increase in oral hypoglycemics dose on most visits. The final A1c value in the intervention group decreased from 11.5% to 9.2%, and in the control group it decreased from 12.2% to 12.1%. This difference between groups was statistically significant. Quality-of-life analyses revealed no significant differences in any of the domains tested between or within groups. No significant changes were noted within or between groups in blood pressure, body weight, serum lipid measurements and renal function parameters.

Kibriya MG et al. (1999) [27] Physicians of the Bangladesh Institute of Research and Rehabilitation in Diabetes Endocrine and Metabolic disorders (BIRDEM) recruited 64 type 2 diabetic patients of "higher-middle class to rich socio-economic class and having completed secondary school certificate level education" to participate in this randomized study and followed them for 18 months. Their aim was to evaluate the cost effectiveness of SMBG in the management of type 2 diabetes in developing countries. All patients received education on diet and how to adjust insulin or oral antidiabetic medications. Patients in the SMBG group were advised to check their blood glucose two to three times a day every two weeks and adjust their medications accordingly if fasting values were >6.0 mmol/L. They were also asked to visit the physician at three month intervals for blood glucose and A1c measurements. Patients in the control group visited the physician at one month intervals and had their antidiabetic regimen modified if needed, based on fasting blood glucose measurements at the monthly visits and A1c values at each three month visit. Cost analysis was performed using conveyance cost, patient wage loss, costs of test strips, glucometer, laboratory tests, and manpower. For the control group, results demonstrated a decrease of 0.43% in A1c after 18 months which was statistically significant. Statistical comparisons between groups were not reported. The SMBG group demonstrated a 1.37% drop in A1c after 18 months which was also significant. Cost analysis revealed comparable results for both groups ($134.55 for the control group vs. $134.75 for the SMBG group). Conclusions were that SMBG with proper diabetes education is a cost effective strategy in the management of type 2 diabetes.

Schwedes U et al. (2002) [29] This study was a randomized multicenter trial that recruited subjects in Germany and Austria and followed them for six months. A total of 250 patients were randomized within blocks of eight to one of two groups: one group used SMBG, kept a blood glucose/eating diary, and received standardized counseling; the control group received only nonstandardized counseling on diet and lifestyle. Two hundred and twenty three patients were included in the final analysis. Patients in the SMBG group were instructed to measure blood glucose six times a day (pre-and postprandially) on two days per week, and to document eating habits and state of well-being. Patients were seen every four weeks. Results showed a statistically significant difference in A1c reduction between the two groups. The control group had a 0.54% reduction of A1c compared to a 1.0% reduction in the SMBG group.

Guerci B et al. (2003) [30] The Auto-Surveillance Intervention Active (ASIA) study out of France followed 689 patients for six months. Patients were randomized to receive either a conventional laboratory work-up based solely on A1c measurements every 12 weeks (control group) or conventional laboratory work-up and SMBG at a frequency of at least six times a week (intervention group). Both groups received counseling on diet and exercise from their general practitioners during five visits throughout the course of the study. At the three month visit, practitioners could modify treatments of their patients based on their A1c value measured at that time. All but three of the patients were on at least one oral antidiabetic drug. Among those, the most widely prescribed drugs were sulfonylureas and biguanides. Results demonstrated a 0.28% absolute greater drop in A1c in the SMBG group as compared to the control group at the end of the study, which was statistically significant. This difference was most pronounced at three months, with a steady state reached in the last three months of the study. The authors concluded that SMBG was associated with better quality of metabolic control than usual recommendations alone in patients with type 2 diabetes. They noted that since no specific instruction for adjusting behavior to the results of SMBG was given to the patients.

Davidson MB et al.(2005) [32] This randomized controlled trial followed 88 patients for six months. Patients in the treatment group were instructed to measure pre- and post-prandial blood glucose levels six days a week. Patients in both groups received dietitian counseling five times during the study. A nurse, who was blinded to whether the patient was in the treatment group or not, followed a detailed algorithm to make her therapeutic decisions. Her goals were to lower fasting glucose concentrations to <130mg/dL by stepwise increases in metformin or a sulfonylurea agent every two weeks, and to achieve an A1c value <7.5%. If the goal A1c was not achieved, a thiazolidinedione was added. Results demonstrated a significant drop in A1c levels of both groups, but no statistically significant difference between the two groups.

Farmer A et al.(2007) [33] This trial randomized 453 patients seen at 48 general practices in London into three groups (usual care, SMBG, SMBG plus training to use results for self care). Patients were included if they had type 2 diabetes, were at least 25 years old at diagnosis, were managed with diet or oral hypoglycemics, had an A1c level greater than or equal to 6.2% at the initial visit, and were able to independently perform daily living activities. Patients in the control group (n=152) received standardized usual care and were seen for A1c measurements once every three months for 12 months. Patients in the less intensive SMBG group (n=150) were instructed to monitor three times a day on two days of every week. In addition to being instructed about self-monitoring, patients in the more intensive SMBG group (n=151) were trained to use the results for self care. Patients in the more intensive group were not instructed to measure blood glucose a set number of times per week, but rather to "explore the effect of different activities... on their blood glucose level." From diaries kept by the patients, those in the more intensive group tested their blood sugar on average six times per week early in the study, but by the end of the 12 months this had decreased to an average of five times per week. Patients in the less intensive group tested their blood sugar on average about five times per week throughout the trial. At three, six, nine, and 12 months no statistically significant differences in A1c levels were found between the three groups.

Key Question #1: Is regular self-monitoring of blood glucose effective in achieving target A1c levels for patients with type 2 diabetes?

Studies of Efficacy

Achieving Target A1c Levels
We identified a single trial that assessed the effect of SMBG (plus counseling and education) in 149 patients in general practice in the Netherlands at meeting target A1c levels. [23] In this study the target A1c level was 8.0%. Prior to the intervention 45 and 41 patients in the in control and intervention arms, respectively, had an A1c values greater than 8%. After the intervention, one patient (2%) and two patients (5%) in the control and intervention arms had A1c values of less than 8% (p=0.6).
Thus there is little evidence to draw a conclusion about the efficacy of SMBG at achieving target A1c levels. We judged the strength of this evidence as very low. [GRADE: Very Low = Any estimate of effect is very uncertain.]

Improving Glycemic Control
While not directly answering this question but certainly relevant to it, is the effect of SMBG on the mean A1c level. All 10 trials reported this outcome. We grouped trials based on the duration of the intervention. The individual and pooled results are shown in Figure 2.

We identified three trials that reported A1c outcomes at three months. [19,25,33] The three trials reported variable results. [19,25] We did not pool the results of these three trials because their results were too heterogeneous, with an I^2 statistic of 67%.

We identified five trials that reported outcomes at about six months. [20,29,30,32,33] Only one trial reported a statistically significant improvement in A1c[30], although a second trial also yielded a statistically significant result after adjusting for baseline difference[29]. The random effects pooled estimate of effect of these five trials was a change in mean A1c value of -0.21% (95% CI: -0.38%, -0.04%). The I^2 statistic for heterogeneity was 0.

We identified five trials that reported outcomes at about one year or longer. [19,23,24,27,33] No study reported a statistically significant difference between groups in the mean A1c value, although two studies reported statistically significant benefits after adjusting for baseline differences in A1c values. [23,27] The random effects pooled estimate of the effect of these five trials was a change in A1c value of -0.15%(95% CI: -0.36%, 0.06%). The I^2 statistic for heterogeneity was 0.

We performed several additional analyses. First we compared studies scores, four or more Delphi items positively (which we called "High quality") with those scoring less than four items positively ("Low quality"). The pooled results showed no statistically significant differences between high and low quality studies.

Figure 2. Analysis of Mean Difference between Control and SMBG Group at Follow-up

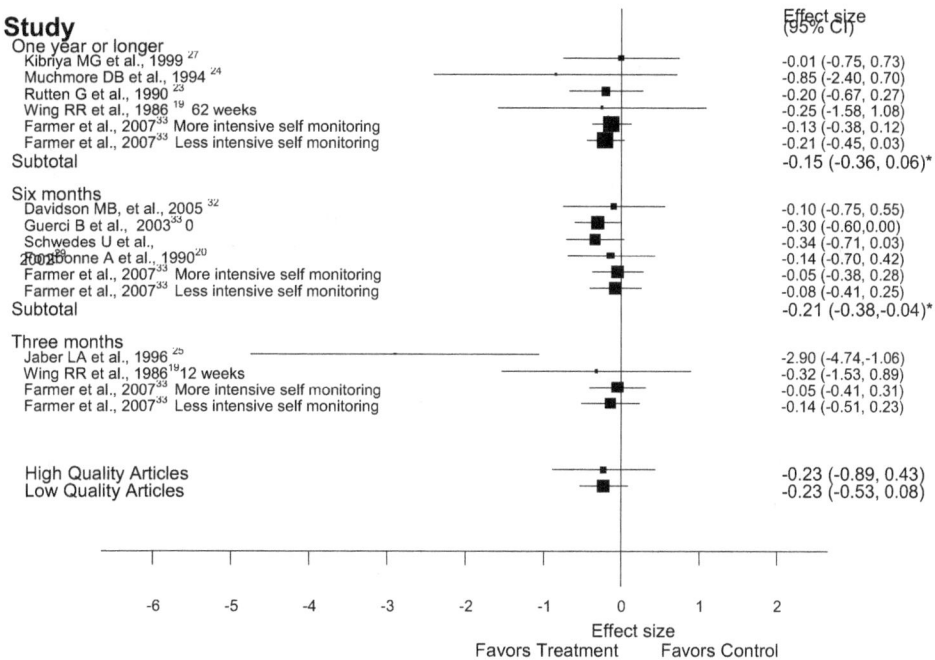

*Subtotal does not include "Farmer et al., 2007 [#1039] Less intensively self monitoring" arm.

We repeated our primary analysis using as the outcome the difference in A1c levels between groups adjusted for baseline A1c levels (whether or not to do such adjusting in the results of an RCT is controversial). When analyzed this way there was much greater heterogeneity between studies, with I^2 statistics of 49% and 75% for studies with six month and 12 month outcomes respectively. However, despite this our primary pooled results were remarkably similar: a modest and statistically significant effect on A1c at six months of 0.19 (compared to a pooled result of 0.21 in the main analysis); and a nonsignificant effect at 12 months. In the difference of difference analysis, high quality studies reported lower estimates of effect than low quality studies, an observation seen in other conditions.[34] This re-analysis supported our primary analysis (Figure 3).

Meta-regression on baseline values of A1c level showed differential effectiveness (p value for difference = 0.05), with higher baseline values of A1c being associated with lesser efficacy of SMBG. Each 1% increase in A1c was associated with a 0.3% decrease in efficacy of SMBG. Thus, indirect evidence suggests that SMBG results in a smaller percent change in A1c for patients with higher baseline values of A1c.

We attempted to identify other components of the intervention or characteristics of the patients associated with greater effectiveness. The trials did not have sufficient similarity in intervention components to permit a meta-regression analysis (See Figure 2). Almost all studies included SMBG and counseling/education, making an assessment of the effect of one without the other impossible, and other intervention components were too sparsely distributed to support meta-regression. Meta-regression using the quality assessment (as either a continuous variable or dichotomous at a threshold value of four) also did not demonstrative differences between results. An analysis of the frequency of SMBG testing is discussed in Key Question #4.

The funnel plot for publication bias is shown in Figure 4. Neither Begg's test nor Eggar's test yielded evidence of unexplained heterogeneity.

Therefore, we found that adding SMBG along with education, counseling, (and some times other components) results in a statistically significant decrease in A1c level of an absolute 0.21% at six months. Results at three months and one year are more variable, although there is a suggestion that this benefit may continue out to at least one year (absolute reduction = -0.15%, 95% CI: -0.36, 0.06). Indirect evidence suggests SMBG maybe less efficacious in subjects with higher baseline A1c values.

We judged the strength of evidence for this outcome as moderate, because individual trials did not in general report significant results and interventions were heterogeneous. [GRADE: Moderate= Further research is likely to have an important impact on our confidence in the estimate of effect and may change the estimate.]

Figure 3. Analysis of Difference of Differences between Control and SMBG Group at Follow-up

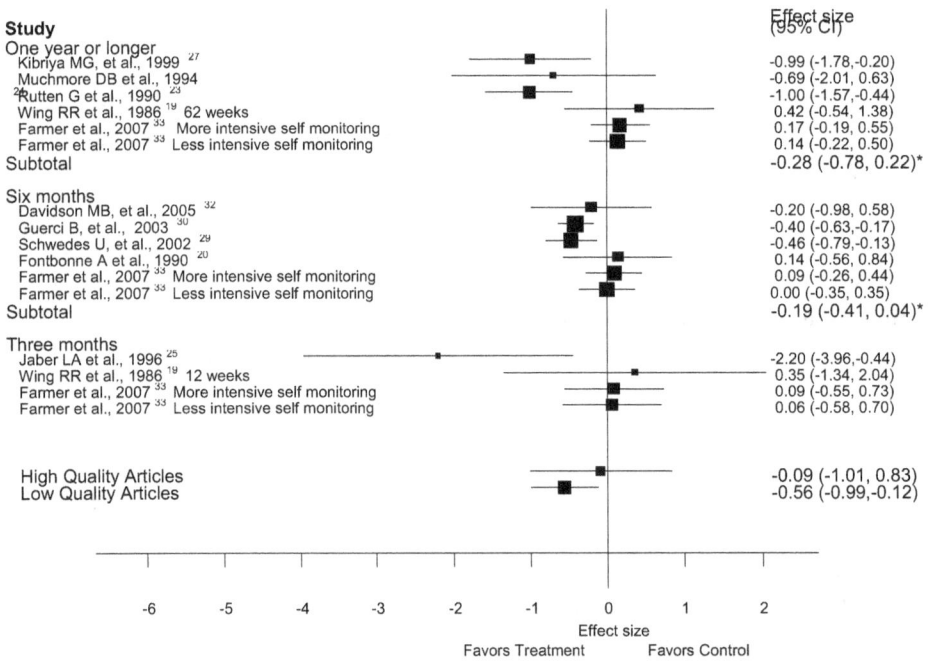

*Subtotal does not include "Farmer et al., 2007 [#1039] Less intensively self monitoring" arm.

Figure 4. Publication Bias for the 10 RCTs

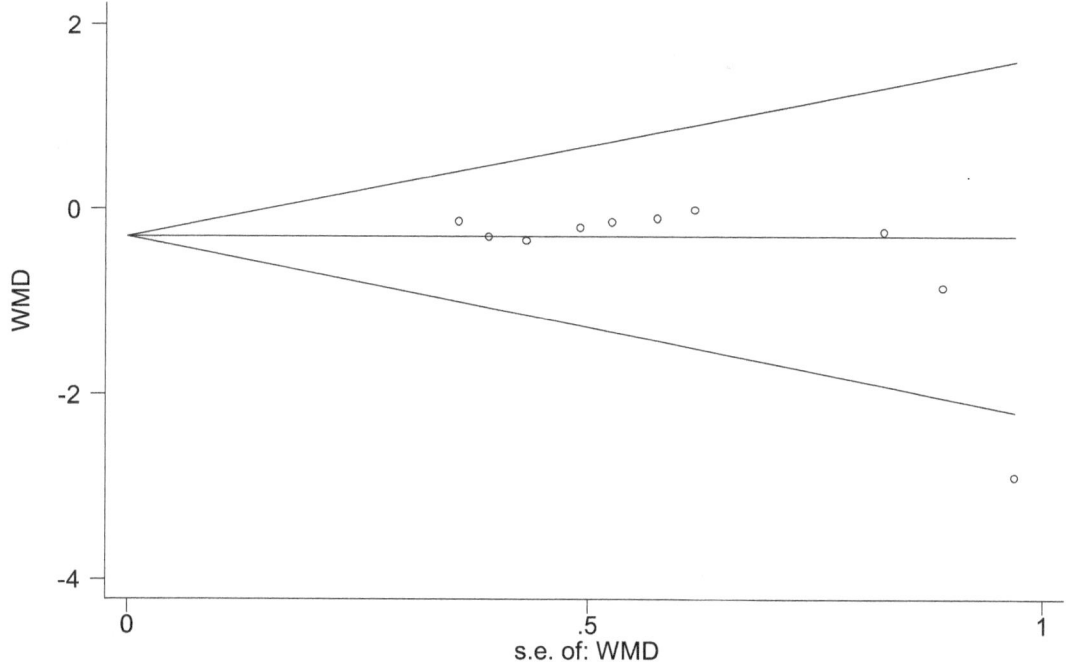

Begg's funnel plot with pseudo 95% confidence limits

Studies of Effectiveness in Veterans

We identified six publications assessing the value of SMBG specifically in Veterans. One publication was an RCT comparing SMBG with urine glucose monitoring, [22] and did not include a comparison with Veterans who did no monitoring. The other five studies were observational in design, mostly retrospective chart reviews that sought to compare a variety of outcomes between Veteran patients receiving supplies for SMBG with those not receiving such supplies. [35-39] Details of all studies are in Table 3.

All studies reported that there was no difference in A1c levels between groups. Although most studies attempted to try and control for baseline differences between patients, the observational study design cannot inform what the A1c values of Veteran patients currently using SMBG would be if they did not receive SMBG supplies. It is possible, for example, that Veterans are selected by their clinicians for receipt of SMBG because they are more difficult to control.

Therefore, the results of the effectiveness studies do not negate the efficacy evidence from RCTs that the addition of SMBG and education can result in a decrease in A1c levels of about 0.3% absolute at six months and up to one year. However, these studies do raise the question of whether Veteran patients are receiving the full possible benefits of SMBG. For example, the RCTs reporting benefit also all included counseling and education. If this is necessary for SMBG to have an effect, one explanation of the difference in the results between the RCTs and the observational studies in veterans is that there is inadequate counseling and education of the Veterans.

We judge the strength of evidence for this outcome as very low because these are observational studies with serious limitations in study quality. [GRADE: Very Low = Any estimate of effect is very uncertain.]

Table 3. Studies of Self-monitoring of Blood Glucose in Veterans

Author/year	Study Design	Patients	SMBG	Duration of Follow-up	Results
Malik RL et al. (1989) [36]	Prospective cohort	16 male Veterans Mean age=62 years Mean duration of DM=8.9years Mean A1c=11.0	"Daily test and adjustment diary" to record SMBG test results and diet changes (average=10 tests/week); 3 4-hour diabetes educational seminars	12 weeks	Improvement in A1c from 11.0 ± 2.9% to 9.9 ± 2.4%, Results reported as not statistically significant.
Newman WP, et al. (1990) [35]	Retrospective cohort	21 Veterans who self-monitored glucose, 17 Veterans who did not Mean duration of DM=17 & 11 years respectively	All patients performing self-monitoring were cared for and taught by the same physician	3 years	No difference in groups in A1c values over time.
Allen BT, et al. (1990) [22]	RCT	61 Veterans with DM without prior SMBG Mean age=58 years Mean A1c=12.0	SMBG versus urine glucose monitoring	6 months	No difference in groups in A1c values at the end of the study (each had 2.0 decrease compared to baseline).
Klein CE, et al. (1993) [37]	Retrospective cohort chart review	229 Veterans, 97%men Mean age=62 years Mean duration of DM=10 years	181 patients performed SMBG	12 months	No difference in mean A1c level between patients using SMBG versus those using urine glucose monitoring.
Rindone JP, et al. (1997) [38]	Retrospective cohort chart review	115 Veterans Mean age=68 years	58 Veterans received Chemstrips	2 years	No difference in mean A1c levels over 2 years between Veterans receiving Chemstrips and those not receiving Chemstrips.
Wen L, et al. (2004) [39]	Retrospective cohort chart & administrative data review	976 Veterans with DM on oral hypoglycemics, 97% men Mean age varied by group between 59 & 66 years A1c levels varied between 6.6 and 7.25	161 Veterans received no Chemstrips, 75 Veterans received Chemstrips in 1 year only, 138 Veterans received Chemstrips in 2 years only, and 602 Veterans received Chemstrips in all 3 years	3 years	No association between use of Chemstrips and mean A1c levels.

DM=Diabetes Mellitus

Key Question #2: Is regular self-monitoring of blood glucose effective in maintaining target A1c levels for patients with type 2 diabetes?

We did not identify any trials that directly assessed this question. Therefore, we draw no conclusion. [GRADE: Very Low = Any estimate of effect is very uncertain.]

Key Question 3: Does regular self-monitoring of blood glucose reduce the frequency of hypoglycemia in patients with type 2 diabetes?

We identified four trials that reported hypoglycemia as an outcome. More details of these trials were presented previously. A brief synopsis of each study follows, with respect to the hypoglycemia outcomes.

Jaber LA et al. (1996) [25] There were 17 reported hypoglycemic reactions in the intervention group and two in the control group. All were rated as mild to moderate, and successfully self-treated. The authors report: "High rate of reported hypoglycemia is partly inherent to the study design and execution. Intervention group patients were repeatedly instructed to and trained on recognition and documentation of hypoglycemia. They were also questioned about the occurrence of these reactions at every clinic visit. Subjects in the control group were not given any specific instructions regarding hypoglycemia and data on its occurrence were collected at the end of the study where capture of this information may have been hindered by the duration of the elapsed time".

Kibriya MG et al. (1999) [27] In this trial the patients in the SMBG group were instructed to perform testing every two weeks, and adjust the dose of anti-diabetic medication accordingly. Control group patients were seen by their doctors on a monthly basis, and had their anti-diabetic treatment modified if needed. During 18 months of follow-up, ten patients in the SMBG intervention group had a total of 17 episodes of hypoglycemia, and five patients from the control group had seven similar episodes. Two patients from the SMBG group needed hospitalization for hyperglycemia compared to none in the control group.

Guerci B et al. (2003) [30] During this trial 78 patients reported at least one episode of hypoglycemia, either symptomatic or asymptomatic: 53(10%) patients in the SMBG group and 25(5%) patients in the control group. These proportions were significantly different due to asymptomatic hypoglycemia alone (P=0.001). There was no serious episode of hypoglycemia reported.

Farmer A et al. (2007) [33] This trial classified hypoglycemia as grade 2 (mild symptoms requiring minor intervention), grade 3 (moderate symptoms requiring immediate third party intervention), and grade 4 (unconscious). Fourteen patients in the control group had at least one grade 2 hypoglycemia episode, compared to 33 patients in the less intensive intervention group and 43 patients in the more intensive intervention group and 43 patients in the more intensive intervention group (p<0.001). One patient in the control group had a grade 3 hypoglycemic episode.

Thus, the limited evidence available indicates that SMBG increases the frequency of recognized hypoglycemia. This is due to an increase in asymptomatic low blood sugar readings, and also an increase in mild-to-moderate symptomatic episodes. There is scant evidence about the effect of SMBG on more clinically significant hypoglycemia. We judge the strength of evidence for SMBG increasing asymptomatic and mildly symptomatic hypoglycemia as moderate. [Moderate = Further research is likely to have an important impact on our confidence in the estimate of effect and may change the estimate.]

Key Question 4: Is there evidence that different frequencies of testing result in differences in improvements in A1c?

We did not identify any study that explicitly tested the effect of different frequency of SMBG on outcomes. This could have been accomplished either as an RCT (randomizing patients to differing frequencies and comparing outcomes) or as an analysis of outcomes within a cohort of patients using SMBG. We therefore were compelled to use an indirect method to examine this question. The indirect method compares the outcomes of studies that vary in the frequency of reported use of SMBG. Indirect methods have only a limited ability to control for other study level differences.

We used meta-regression to assess the effect of the reported frequency of SMBG use in the RCTs (measured as times/week) on differences in A1c level compared to control. No association was found (p=0.99). Therefore we draw no conclusion about the effect of frequency of SMBG monitoring on A1c values, and judge the strength of the evidence to be very low. [GRADE: Very Low = Any estimate of effect is very uncertain.]

SUMMARY AND DISCUSSION

In this chapter, we describe the limitations of our review and meta-analysis and then present our conclusions. We also discuss the implications of our findings for future research.

Limitations

Publication Bias

Our literature search procedures were extensive and included all articles identified in prior reviews plus additional articles. Our formal tests for publication bias did not indicate the presence of possible publication bias but such tests do not exclude the possibility that such bias exists. Therefore, readers are cautioned about this possibility.

Study Quality

An important limitation common to systematic reviews is the quality of the original studies. Recent attempts to define elements of study design and execution that are related to bias have shown that in many cases, such efforts are not reproducible and do not distinguish study results based on bias. Therefore, the current approach is to avoid rejecting studies or using quality criteria to adjust the meta-analysis results. We did use the Delphi list[10] as a descriptive measure of quality. As there is a lack of empirical evidence regarding study characteristics and their relationship to bias, we did not attempt to use other criteria. Other aspects of the design and execution of a trial may be related to bias, but we do not yet have good measures of these elements. The sensitivity analysis of our main result did not yield any suggestion that the quality of the trials influenced our findings in a significant way.

Heterogeneity

While there were some differences in the population being assessed and the number of times and timing of SMBG recommended, the most important heterogeneity in this review was the differing intervention components added to SMBG and the difference in the recommendations for frequency of SMBG testing, provider interaction or algorithm to adjust medications, and intensity of education. While the statistical test for heterogeneity was not significant for six months and 12 month outcomes, this test has low power and does not preclude substantial heterogeneity among studies. There were too few studies to be able to support meta-regression to assess the relative effectiveness of these differences.

Applicability of Findings

Green & Glasgow[40] provide a framework for evaluating the relevance, generalization, and applicability of research. Their framework includes assessing the participation rate, the intended target population, the representativeness of the setting, the representativeness of the individuals, and evaluating information about implementation and assessment of outcomes. As these data are rarely reported in the studies we reviewed, conclusions about applicability are necessarily weak. Furthermore, none of the trials assessed VA patients or VA core delivery systems. The observational studies done in VA did not report results compatible with SMBG being an effective intervention; however RCTs are generally preferred to observational studies when making estimates of efficacy and effectiveness.

Conclusions

With the above limitations in mind, we reached the conclusions displayed below.

KEY QUESTION #1: Is regular SMBG effective in achieving target A1c levels for patients with type 2 diabetes?

Studies of Efficacy
Achieving Target A1c Levels
There is little evidence to draw a conclusion about the effect of SMBG at achieving target A1c levels. We judged the strength of this evidence as very low. [GRADE: Very Low = Any estimate of effect is very uncertain.]

Improving Glycemic Control
We found that adding SMBG along with education, counseling, (and some times other components) results in a statistically significant decrease in A1c level of an absolute 0.21% at six months. Results at three months and one year are more variable, although there is a suggestion that this benefit may continue out to at least one year.

We judged the strength of evidence for this outcome as moderate, because individual trials did not in general report significant results and interventions were heterogeneous. [GRADE: Moderate= Further research is likely to have an important impact on our confidence in the estimate of effect and may change the estimate.]

Studies of Effectiveness in Veterans
Five observational studies of SMBG effectiveness in Veteran populations did not report statistically significant improvements in glycemic control. The results of the studies with Veterans do not negate the evidence from RCTs that the addition of SMBG and education can result in a decrease in A1c levels of about 0.3% absolute at six months and up to one year. However, these studies do raise the question of whether veteran patients are receiving the full possible benefits of SMBG. [GRADE: Very Low = Any estimate of effect is very uncertain.]

KEY QUESTION #2: Is regular SMBG effective in maintaining target A1c levels for patients with type 2 diabetes?

We did not identify any trials that directly assessed this question. Therefore, we draw no conclusion. [GRADE: Very Low = Any estimate of effect is very uncertain.]

KEY QUESTION #3: Does regular SMBG reduce the frequency of hypoglycemia in patients with type 2 diabetes?

The limited evidence available indicates that SMBG increases the frequency of recognized hypoglycemia. This is due to an increase in asymptomatic low blood sugar readings, and also an increase in mild-to-moderate symptomatic episodes. There is scant evidence about the effect of SMBG on more clinically significant hypoglycemia. We judge the strength of evidence for

SMBG increasing asymptomatic and mildly symptomatic hypoglycemia as moderate. [Moderate = Further research is likely to have an important impact on our confidence in the estimate of effect and may change the estimate.]

KEY QUESTION #4: Is there evidence that different frequencies of testing result in differences in improvements in A1c?

We used meta-regression to assess the effect of the reported frequency of SMBG use in the RCTs (measures as times/week) on differences in A1c level compared to control. No association was found (p=0.99). Therefore we draw no conclusion about the effect of frequency of SMBG monitoring on A1c values, and judge the strength of the evidence to be very low. [GRADE: Very Low = Any estimate of effect is very uncertain.]

FUTURE RESEARCH

Our review of existing data support the short term beneficial effect of SMBG on A1c levels in the context of a clinical trial. Although improvement in A1c is modest, it is approximately equivalent to that achieved with diabetes education interventions. [41]Whether the benefit extends beyond six months is questionable.

However, observational studies in the VA do not report differences in A1c levels between Veterans using or not using SMBG supplies. This raises the question about implementation: more research is needed to understand if implementation of SMBG in a typical VA clinic setting is sufficient for Veterans to receive the full benefit reported in clinical trials.

In particular, it would be worthwhile to conduct studies in VA of "enhanced" SMBG versus usual care SMBG, with "enhanced" computer-based or nurse case-management or being Health Buddy or My Healthe Vet facilitated implementation of SMBG. This would more closely approximate the study question of interest today. New studies would also be able to account for improvements in SMBG technology (meters, strips, etc.) over time.

Additionally, data are needed about the cost-effectiveness of SMBG in a VA setting.

The evidence is insufficient to draw conclusions about which components of SMBG (additional-education, algorithms or other techniques to adjust medication) and frequency of testing are most associated with better results. More research is needed, and again we note that it should consider incorporation of methods for enhancing SMBG effectiveness. Additionally the impact of SMBG on medication adherence should be evaluated.

REFERENCE LIST

1. WHO media centre. Diabetes. 2006. 2001.

2. National Diabetes Information Clearinghouse. National Diabetes Statistics. 2005. 2007.

3. Stratton IM, Adler AI, Neil HA, Matthews DR, Manley SE, Cull CA, et al. Association of glycaemia with macrovascular and microvascular complications of type 2 diabetes (UKPDS 35): prospective observational study. BMJ 2000; 321:405-12.

4. Faas A, Schellevis FG, Van Eijk JT. The efficacy of self-monitoring of blood glucose in NIDDM subjects. A criteria-based literature review. Diabetes Care 1997; 20:1482-6.

5. Coster S, Gulliford MC, Seed PT, Powrie JK, Swaminathan R. Self-monitoring in Type 2 diabetes mellitus: a meta-analysis. Diabet Med 2000; 17:755-61.

6. Welschen LM, Bloemendal E, Nijpels G, Dekker JM, Heine RJ, Stalman WA, et al. Self-monitoring of blood glucose in patients with type 2 diabetes who are not using insulin: a systematic review. Diabetes Care 2005; 28:1510-7.

7. Balk E, Teplinsky E, Trikalinos T, Chew P, Chung M, Pittas A. 20 Date of Publication>; Maryland: Agency for Healthcare Research and Quality.

8. Jansen JP. Self-monitoring of glucose in type 2 diabetes mellitus: a Bayesian meta-analysis of direct and indirect comparisons. Curr Med Res Opin 2006; 22:671-81.

9. Furukawa TA, Barbui C, Cipriani A, Brambilla P, Watanabe N. Imputing missing standard deviations in meta-analyses can provide accurate results. J Clin Epidemiol 2006; 59:7-

10. Verhagen AP, de Vet HC, de Bie RA, Kessels AG, Boers M, Bouter LM, et al. The Delphi list: a criteria list for quality assessment of randomized clinical trials for conducting systematic reviews developed by Delphi consensus. J Clin Epidemiol 1998; 51:1235-41.

11. Suttorp M, Shekelle P, van Tulder M, Morton S, Bouter L. Cochran Back Group Quality Item and Bias in Back Pain Trials. Abstract.

12. Ray JW, Shadish WR. How interchangeable are different estimators of effect size? J Consult Clin Psychol 1996; 64:1316-25.

13. DerSimonian R, Laird N. Meta-analysis in clinical trials. Control Clin Trials 1986; 7:177-88.

14. Berkey CS, Hoaglin DC, Mosteller F, Colditz GA. A random-effects regression model for meta-analysis. Stat Med 1995; 14:395-411.

15. Hedges LV, Olkin I. Statistical Methods for Meta-Analysis. San Diego, CA: Academic Press Inc, 1985.

16. Higgins JP, Thompson SG, Deeks JJ, Altman DG. Measuring inconsistency in meta-analyses. BMJ 2003; 327:557-60.

17. Stata Statistical Software Manual [computer program]. 2006; ed.

18. Atkins D, Best D, Briss PA, Eccles M, Falck-Ytter Y, Flottorp S, et al. Grading quality of evidence and strength of recommendations. BMJ 2004; 328:1490

19. Wing RR, Epstein LH, Nowalk MP, Scott N, Koeske R, Hagg S. Does self-monitoring of blood glucose levels improve dietary compliance for obese patients with type II diabetes? Am J Med 1986; 81:830-6.

20. Fontbonne A, Billault B, Acosta M, Percheron C, Varenne P, Besse A, et al. Is glucose self-monitoring beneficial in non-insulin-treated diabetic patients? Results of a randomized comparative trial. Diabete Metab 1989; 15:255-60.

21. Estey AL, Tan MH, Mann K. Follow-up intervention: its effect on compliance behavior to a diabetes regimen. Diabetes Educ 1990; 16:291-5.

22. Allen BT, DeLong ER, Feussner JR. Impact of glucose self-monitoring on non-insulin-treated patients with type II diabetes mellitus. Randomized controlled trial comparing blood and urine testing. Diabetes Care 1990; 13:1044-50.

23. Rutten G, van Eijk J, de Nobel E, Beek M, van der Velden H. Feasibility and effects of a diabetes type II protocol with blood glucose self-monitoring in general practice. Fam Pract 1990; 7:273-8.

24. Muchmore DB, Springer J, Miller M. Self-monitoring of blood glucose in overweight type 2 diabetic patients. Acta Diabetol 1994; 31:215-9.

25. Jaber LA, Halapy H, Fernet M, Tummalapalli S, Diwakaran H. Evaluation of a pharmaceutical care model on diabetes management. Ann Pharmacother 1996; 30:238-43.

26. Miles P, Everett J, Murphy J, Kerr D. Comparison of blood or urine testing by patients with newly diagnosed non-insulin dependent diabetes: patient survey after randomised crossover trial. BMJ 1997; 315:348-9.

27. Kibriya MG, Ali L, Banik NG, Khan AK. Home monitoring of blood glucose (HMBG) in Type-2 diabetes mellitus in a developing country. Diabetes Res Clin Pract 1999; 46:253-7.

28. Brown SA, Garcia AA, Kouzekanani K, Hanis CL. Culturally competent diabetes self-management education for Mexican Americans: the Starr County border health initiative. Diabetes Care 2002; 25:259-68.

29. Schwedes U, Siebolds M, Mertes G. Meal-related structured self-monitoring of blood glucose: effect on diabetes control in non-insulin-treated type 2 diabetic patients. Diabetes Care 2002; 25:1928-32.

30. Guerci B, Drouin P, Grange V, Bougneres P, Fontaine P, Kerlan V, et al. Self-monitoring of blood glucose significantly improves metabolic control in patients with type 2 diabetes mellitus: the Auto-Surveillance Intervention Active (ASIA) study. Diabetes Metab 2003; 29:587-94.

31. Kwon HS, Cho JH, Kim HS, Song BR, Ko SH, Lee JM, et al. Establishment of blood glucose monitoring system using the internet. Diabetes Care 2004; 27:478-83.

32. Davidson MB, Castellanos M, Kain D, Duran P. The effect of self monitoring of blood glucose concentrations on glycated hemoglobin levels in diabetic patients not taking insulin: a blinded, randomized trial. Am J Med 2005; 118:422-5.

33. Farmer A, Wade A, Goyder E, Yudkin P, French D, Craven A, et al. Impact of self monitoring of blood glucose in the management of patients with non-insulin treated diabetes: open parallel group randomised trial. BMJ 2007;

34. Moher D, Pham B, Jones A, Cook DJ, Jadad AR, Moher M, et al. Does quality of reports of randomised trials affect estimates of intervention efficacy reported in meta-analyses? Lancet 1998; 352:609-13.

35. Newman WP, Laqua D, Engelbrecht D. Impact of glucose self-monitoring on glycohemoglobin values in a veteran population. Arch Intern Med 1990; 150:107-10.

36. Malik RL, Horwitz DL, McNabb WL, Takaki ET, Hawkins HA, Keys AG, et al. Adjustment of caloric intake based on self-monitoring in noninsulin-dependent diabetes mellitus: development and feasibility. J Am Diet Assoc 1989; 89:960-1.

37. Klein CE, Oboler SK, Prochazka A, Oboler S, Frank M, Glugla M, et al. Home blood glucose monitoring: effectiveness in a general population of patients who have non-insulin-dependent diabetes mellitus. J Gen Intern Med 1993; 8:597-601.

38. Rindone JP, Austin M, Luchesi J. Effect of home blood glucose monitoring on the management of patients with non-insulin dependent diabetes mellitus in the primary care setting. Am J Manag Care 1997; 3:1335-8.

39. Williams GC, McGregor H, Zeldman A, Freedman ZR, Deci EL, Elder D. Promoting glycemic control through diabetes self-management: evaluating a patient activation intervention. Patient Educ Couns 2005; 56:28-34.

40. Green LW, Glasgow RE. Evaluating the relevance, generalization, and applicability of research: issues in external validation and translation methodology. Eval Health Prof 2006; 29:126-53.

41. Norris SL, Lau J, Smith SJ, Schmid CH, Engelgau MM. Self-management education for adults with type 2 diabetes: a meta-analysis of the effect on glycemic control. Diabetes Care 2002; 25:1159-71.

APPENDIX A. DATA COLLECTION FORMS

Article ID   **Reviewers:**   **Assigned on:**

Citation:

First Author:_____

Complete Q7 & Q8 on ALL forms

1. Is the study a test of efficacy or effectiveness of SMBG alone or as part of a multi-component intervention?
   (Check all that apply)
   Alone……………………………….☐
   Multi-component………………..….☐
   No…………………………………...☐ **(STOP)**

2. Study design
   (Circle one)
   RCT/CCT……………………….....…1
   Review article: systematic or M-A....2
   Observational Study (cohort,
   case control, etc)……………3 **(STOP)**
   Review article: Not systematic……..4 **(STOP)**
   Review article: letter, editorial,
   other syst review………….. 5 **(STOP)**
   Other……………………………...6 **(STOP)**

2a. Is this a crossover study?
   (Circle one)
   Yes…………………………………1
   No…………………………………..0

3. Is A1c reported as an outcome?
   (Circle one)
   Yes…………………………………1
   No…………………………………..0

4. Is hypoglycemia reported as an outcome?
   (Circle one)
   Yes…………………………………1
   No…………………………………..0

5. Is the frequency of SMBG testing reported?
   (Circle one)
   Yes…………………………………1
   No…………………………………..0

6. If RCT/CCT or observational study, what is the duration of the follow up?
   (Circle one)
   < 12 weeks/not an RCT/CCT or
   observational study…………0 **(STOP)**
   12 weeks or greater ……………….1
   If >=12 wks, write in the duration

Duration	**Units**	**Units**
___ ___ ___	___ ___	01. Days 04. Years 02. Weeks 05. NR 03. Months

7. If this article meets no other criterion, should it be saved for background?
   (Circle one)
   Yes…………………………………1
   No…………………………………..0

8. Are any of the subjects identified as Veterans?
   (Circle one)
   Yes…………………………………1
   No…………………………………..0

Notes

VA Self-Monitoring of Blood Glucose Project-Detailed Review Form

FINAL 12-14-06

Article ID: Reviewer:

First Author:
          (Last Name Only)

Study Number: _____ of _____   Description: _____
          (Enter '1 of 1' if only one)   (if more than one **study**)

1. Do you think that this article might include the same data as another study?

          (CIRCLE ONE)
   Yes....................................1
   No.....................................2
          If YES enter IDs:
          ID(s) : _____

2. Design: (CIRCLE ONE)
   RCT...................................1
   CCT...................................2
   Other design......................3   (STOP)

3. Is the study described as randomized?   (CIRCLE ONE)
   Yes....................................1
   No.....................................2

4. If the study was randomized, was method of randomization appropriate?   (CIRCLE ONE)
   Yes....................................1
   No.....................................2
   Method not described............8
   Not applicable (not randomized) 9

5. Is the study described (with respect to SMBG)as: (CIRCLE ONE)
   Double blind.......................1
   Single blind, patient.............2
   Single blind, outcome assessment 3
   Single blind, not described.....4
   Open..................................5
   Blinding not described............8
   Not applicable.....................9

6. If reported, was the method of double blinding appropriate?   (CIRCLE ONE)
   Yes.....1..............................1
   No.......................................2
   Double blinding method not described..........8
   Not applicable........................(9)

7. If study was randomized, did the method of randomization provide for concealment of allocation?   (CIRCLE ONE)
   Yes....................................1
   No.....................................2
   Concealment not described........8
   Not applicable (not randomized) 9

8. Are withdrawals (W) and dropouts (D) described?   (CIRCLE ONE)
   Yes, reason described for **all** W and D.......1
   Yes, reason described for **some** W and D.......2
   Not described........................8
   Not applicable.......................9

9. Is the study a cross-over study design?   (CIRCLE ONE)
   Yes....................................1
   No.....................................2

10. Sample size: (Enter 999 for not reported)

   Enrolled: _____ _____ _____
   Followed-up/analyzed: _____ _____ _____

VA Self-Monitoring of Blood Glucose Project-Detailed Review Form

11. What were the characteristics of the patient population?

A. Demographics:

% women = _____

(CHECK ALL THAT APPLY)

Caucasian .... ☐
African Ancestry .... ☐
Hispanic .... ☐

Other (Specify: _____) .... ☐

Demographics not reported .... ☐

If yes, please enter the following: **Weight** **Units**

Mean weight .... _____ _____

Median weight .... _____ _____

Weight Range .... _____ to _____ _____

Units
1. kilograms
2. pounds
3. NA
4. ND
999. NR

15. Was duration of diabetes reported?

(CIRCLE ONE)

Yes 1
No 0

If yes, please enter the following: **Time** **Units**

Mean time .... _____ _____

Median time .... _____ _____

Time Range .... _____ to _____ _____

Units
1. Hour   5. Year
2. Day   8. ND
3. Week   9. NA
4. Month   999. NR

12. What was reported for the following questions regarding subjects' ages? (Enter number 999 for not reported)

Mean Age .... _____

Median Age .... _____

Age Range .... _____ to _____

13. Was BMI reported?

(CIRCLE ONE)

Yes 1
No 2

If yes, please enter the following: (Enter number 999 for not reported)

Mean BMI .... _____

Median BMI .... _____

BMI Range .... _____ to _____

14. Was weight reported?

(CIRCLE ONE)

Yes 1
No 2

16. Which of the following co-morbidities were reported on:

(CHECK ALL THAT APPLY)

Myocardial infarction .... ☐
CongestiveHeart Failure .... ☐
Peripheral Vascular disease .... ☐

Cerebrovascular disease .... ☐
Dementia .... ☐
Chronic pulmonary disease .... ☐

Rheumatologic disease .... ☐
Peptic ulcer disease .... ☐
Mild liver disease .... ☐
Hemiplegia or paraplegia .... ☐

Renal disease .... ☐
Malignancy, leukemia, lymphoma .... ☐
Moderate-severe liver disease .... 1 ☐
AIDS .... 2 ☐

VA Self-Monitoring of Blood Glucose Project-Detailed Review Form

Enter sample size and intervention/exposure data for each arm beginning with CONTROL/USUAL CARE for arm 1, then in order of first mention.
For observational studies answer only columns denoted with asterisks (*).

Arm/Group	Sample size *	Components * (check all that apply)	Total # of Visits	Frequency of SMBG	Number of Days per week	Duration of * treatment	Units *	Co-therapies(s)
1	P ___ PY ___ CNTRL ___ N ENTERING ___ — CASES ___ N COMPLETING ___	SMBG ☐ Dietician ☐ Pt Control ☐ Not Reported ☐ — Exercise ☐ Other ☐ Not applicable ☐ — Diabetes counseling/Education ☐	___	**Control**	___	___	___	___
2	P ___ PY ___ CNTRL ___ N ENTERING ___ — CASES ___ N COMPLETING ___	SMBG ☐ Dietician ☐ Pt Control ☐ Not Reported ☐ — Exercise ☐ Other ☐ Not applicable ☐ — Diabetes counseling/Education ☐	___	GD ☐ BID ☐ TID ☐ QID ☐ PP ☐ Other ☐ Before/After meals ☐ NR ☐	___	___	___	___
3	P ___ PY ___ CNTRL ___ N ENTERING ___ — CASES ___ N COMPLETING ___	SMBG ☐ Dietician ☐ Pt Control ☐ Not Reported ☐ — Exercise ☐ Other ☐ Not applicable ☐ — Diabetes counseling/Education ☐	___	GD ☐ BID ☐ TID ☐ QID ☐ PP ☐ Other ☐ Before/After meals ☐ NR ☐		___	___	___
4	P ___ PY ___ CNTRL ___ N ENTERING ___ — CASES ___ N COMPLETING ___	SMBG ☐ Dietician ☐ Pt Control ☐ Not Reported ☐ — Exercise ☐ Other ☐ Not applicable ☐ — Diabetes counseling/Education ☐	___	GD ☐ BID ☐ TID ☐ QID ☐ PP ☐ Other ☐ Before/After meals ☐ NR ☐	___	___	___	___
	Enter a number for N entering and N completing or enter 9999 if not reported. If observational study, circle appropriate unit of measurement: P Persons PY People years CNTRL Control CASES Cases		Enter # of visits or contact s		Enter a number 997. Variable 998. ND 999. NA	Enter a number 997. Variable 998. ND 999. NA	Enter a number 1.Hour 2.Day 3.Week 4.Month 5.Year 8.ND, 9. NA	

VA Male OP Project-Detailed Review Form- Diagnostic Studies

Outcomes

17. Please check the type of outcomes measured. For case control enter the outcome that defines the study:

(CHECK ALL THAT APPLY)

	Units	
1. Hour	5. Year	
2. Day	8. ND	
3. Week	9. NA	
4. Month	999. NR	

HbA1c .... ☐

Fasting glucose ....

Fructose .... ☐

BMI/Weight loss .... ☐

Fast v. meal glucose .... ☐

Health related quality of life ... ☐

Adverse Events

19. Were any of the following adverse events mentioned?

(Check all that apply)

Hypoglycemia .... ☐

Other adverse events .... ☐

No Adverse events .... ☐

Not described .... ☐

Not applicable .... ☐

Evaluation

18. When, relative to the start of the intervention, were outcomes reported?

(Enter the number/code in the appropriate box)

	Control		Intervention	
	Number	Units	Number	Units
1st follow-up				
2nd follow-up				
3rd follow-up				
4th follow-up				
5th follow-up				
6th follow-up				
Additional follow-ups				

20.　　Is there a reference that needs to be checked?

(Circle one)

Yes 1

No 2

If YES, which one(s) : _____

(Enter reference # and/or author or 9999 if don't know.)

SMBG Project- Randomized Controlled Trials Quality Measurement

Article ID: _____   Reviewer:

First Author: _____

1. Treatment Allocation
a. Was a method of randomization performed?
Yes .... ☐
No .... ☐
Don't know .... ☐

b. Was the treatment allocation concealed?
Yes .... ☐
No .... ☐
Don't know .... ☐

2. Were the groups similar at baseline regarding the most important prognostic indicators?
Yes .... ☐
No .... ☐
Don't know .... ☐

3. Were the eligibility criteria specified?
Yes .... ☐
No .... ☐
Don't know .... ☐

4. Was the outcome assessor blinded?
Yes .... ☐
No .... ☐
Don't know .... ☐

5. Was the care provider blinded?
Yes .... ☐
No .... ☐
Don't know .... ☐

6. Was the patient blinded?
Yes .... ☐
No .... ☐
Don't know .... ☐

7. Were point estimates and measures of variability presented for the primary outcome measures?
Yes .... ☐
No .... ☐
Don't know .... ☐

8. Did the analysis include an intention-to-treat analysis?
Yes .... ☐
No .... ☐
Don't know .... ☐

APPENDIX B. PEER REVIEW COMMENTS TABLE

Peer Review Comments Table 1.

Reviewer	Section	Comment	Change
Pogach	Background	The investigators frame the background in terms of targets and measures. I would suggest that the background by Guerci in the ASIA study frames the question better: "Theoretically, SMBG can improve compliance with recommendations on diet and exercise and medication regimens. The American Diabetes Association has recommended that the optimal frequency of SMBG for patients with type 2 diabetes should be adequate to facilitate reaching glucose goals. This hypothesis is based on the fact that lifestyle changes are facilitated by SMBG. Under these conditions, we should expect an improvement of glycemic control SMBG increases patient management costs, and because of the high prevalence of type 2 diabetes, efforts to establish the efficacy of SMBG in type 2 diabetes mellitus are of greater relevance."	This suggested change was made, however, reference to targets was kept in this revision as the key questions from VA concern targets and not general improvements in glycemic control.
Pogach	Background	If the investigators want to include a discussion of targets, their reliance on ADA Clinical Practice Recommendations is incomplete, and needs to take into account other guidelines and be more complete in describing the ADA recommendations. The authors frame the ADA recommendations to bias the reviewer towards tight control for most. "The Association (ADA) recommends an A1c goal of <7% for "patients in general" but adds that, "for the individual patient," intensive therapy to achieve an A1c as close to normal (<6%) without hypoglycemia is the goal, although the latter recommendation is based on weaker or incomplete evidence.4 ". To be evidence explicit and transparent, the investigators need to note (to be evidence explicit) that multiple guidelines, including the ADA, American Geriatric Society, and VHA-DOD discuss the need for less stringent targets based upon life expectancy (AGS and VA) or age (ADA >65 years of age), comorbid conditions, and side effects (including hypoglycemia). The ADA "in general" thus refers to individuals who are younger without contraindications. Moreover, the NHLBI study permits an A1c between 7.0-7.9%(expected mean 7.5%) in the control group.	We deemphasized the focus about targets and the ADA, but retained the text about VA performance measures as targets, since the key questions given to us by VA concern efficacy at achieving target glycemic control levels.
Aron	Introduction	This evidence review is being performed by VA. Therefore, it is quite surprising that the recommendations of the American Diabetes Association are so prominently stated. The recent article in the New York Times related to conflicts of interest in determining performance measures should give us pause. I realize that this is in the introduction and meant to provide context, but I would rather have seen studies cited, e.g., DCCT and UKPDS rather than the ADA (or any other advocacy organization).	Text about ADA has been deemphasized.
Pogach	Background	I don't understand why performance measurement is pertinent to the introduction. Only NCQA recommends public reporting for A1c <7% (see Pogach, Engelgau, Aron JAMA 2007). Thus, I would recommend removing references to performance measures as being not relevant.	The text regarding performance measures is retained because VA's questions to us were framed in terms of target levels.
Aron	Study Identification/ Study Selection	Some of the criteria for study inclusion were not explicit. I am referring here specifically to the statement that studies not included in other meta-analyses/reviews were included in this one. The reasons why are not included.	The reasons were indicated in Table 1, and no change was made in the text.
Pogach	Study Identification/ Study Selection	I am not satisfied with the investigators' explanation that "we included studies rejected by Balk and/or by Welschen for a variety of reasons (italics mine)".	
Pogach	Study Identification/ Study Selection	If the investigators believe that their inclusion is still justified, in contrast to the AHRQ Evidence Synthesis (Balk report) the investigators should provide an explicit explanation of the reasons why they disagreed.	
Pogach	Study Identification/ Study Selection	The investigators frame the meta-analysis by noting that it is to address SMBG in individuals on oral hypo-glycemic medications. It is unclear to me whether the Kwan study included individuals on insulin; the Cho study did include 7 out of 40 control groups on insulin (4 insulin only) and 11 of 40 intervention group (6 insulin only). If these studies are included, this needs to be noted as a limitation of generalization of the study findings. In addition, the willingness and ability to use the internet to download meter results may prevent generalization to other populations with lower Socio-economic position.	We agree and the articles by Cho and Kwon were removed from the analysis.
Aron	Study Identification/ Study Selection	P17. "Initial screening of the articles resulted in 13 RCTs that measured the effect of SMBG compared to a group not receiving SMBG and monitored A1c levels with at least three months of follow-up. Two were excluded; one because the trial presented duplicate data, the other because the trial compared a control group of SMBG to an intervention group of SMBG plus other components. (Figure 1)" Unfortunately, this is not the case. The Cho study states: "We performed a diabetes education program again to standardize every patient's education for diabetes management and the method and frequency of self-monitoring of blood glucose (SMBG) according to glucose control." The control group used SMBG. The only difference was that the experimental group had the internet intervention. Why is this study included?	

Peer Review Comments Table 1. Continued

Reviewer	Section	Comment	Change
Pogach	Study Identification/Study Selection	The investigators note that "Initial screening of the articles resulted in 13 RCTs that measured the effect of SMBG compared to a group not receiving SMBG and monitored A1c levels with at least three months of follow-up. Two were excluded; one because the trial presented duplicate data, the other because the trial compared a control group of SMBG to an intervention group of SMBG plus other components. (Figure 1)." By these criteria, the Kwon (2004) and Cho (2006) articles should be excluded, since the control group and intervention group each received the same number of monitoring strips and received the same instructions on monitoring. The intervention being tested was therefore the "Internet Based Blood Glucose Monitoring System", which essentially increased the frequency of access to the diabetes team; electronic case management in a sense. It's my perspective that the investigators are obligated to remove these studies from the main analysis.	We agree and the articles by Cho and Kwon were removed from the analysis.
Pogach	Study Identification/Study Selection	The investigators note that "Eligible study designs included controlled clinical trials, RCTs, and systematic reviews/meta-analyses. Observational studies, case reports, non-systematic reviews, letters to the editor and other similar contributions were excluded." This review separately comments on observational studies done in veterans, but not observational studies of non-veterans. The investigators need to be consistent; either remove them or separately discuss all observational studies. I suggest excluding them as not being relevant to the meta-analysis as defined. In addition, the investigators, in their criteria for inclusion, do not include observational studies. None the less, they include older retrospective VA studies. If they choose to include VA studies, they should modify their inclusion/exclusion criteria to include others. Otherwise (and given that meta-analyses of RCTs have significant limitations as well), I would exclude them.	We have revised the methods and results to indicate that the observational studies in veterans were searched for and reported on as evidence regarding the effectiveness of SMBG in the VA patient population and delivery system, as opposed to the efficacy evidence from RCTs.
Aron	Study Identification/Study Selection	P13 "Eligible study designs included controlled clinical trials, RCTs, and systematic reviews/meta-analyses. Observational studies, case reports, non-systematic reviews, letters to the editor and other similar contributions were excluded." However, in discussing studies in veterans, observational studies were included. It is not clear why they were included here and not elsewhere. The reasons should be made explicit. That also raises the question about using observational studies in non-veterans.	
Aron	Study Identification/Study Selection	Inconsistencies aside, it is an interesting philosophical issue what the appropriate control group should be in studies like this. Individuals with diabetes have free access to SMBG, i.e., can do it without a prescription. What is usual care in this regard?	We agree this is an interesting question. We agree that the Cho and Kwon studies aren't comparing SMBG to no SMBG, so as indicated above, we deleted these. We interpreted VA's main interest as SMBG vs. no SMBG at all.
Pogach	Data Synthesis	A significant positive aspect of this study is to adjust for baseline A1c. This is welcome, and should be commented on in more detail (see also data synthesis).	We have added text about this.
Pogach	Data Synthesis	The reviewer's perspective is that adjusting for baseline HbA1c is an appropriate consideration and can be defended (see Bloomgarden Z et al Lower Baseline Glycemia Reduces Apparent Oral Agent Glucose-Lowering Efficacy: A meta-regression analysis Diabetes Care 2006 29: 2137-2139. This should be commented upon in greater detail.	
Aron	Data Synthesis	It is an interesting issue whether or not to adjust for baseline A1c. I would have liked to see both adjusted and unadjusted analyses.	Only unadjusted pooled results are presented in Figure 2. Figure 3 presents the pooled result of studies adjusting for baseline levels of A1c at the individual study level. The meta-regression analysis assesses the relationship between baseline A1c and efficacy of SMBG. So all three kinds of analyses are already included in the report - unadjusted, adjusted at the individual study level, and adjusted at the pooled analyses level.

Peer Review Comments Table 1. Continued

Reviewer	Section	Comment	Change
Aron	Conclusions	To reiterate, it is not clear why observational studies are included and I don't see how one can draw the conclusion that veteran patients may not be receiving the full possible benefits of SMBG. I happen to agree with the conclusion, but that comes more from my experience in clinic than from these studies.	The reason for including observational VA studies has now been made clear.
Pogach	Conclusions	In multiple sections of the report the investigators state that "The results of the studies with Veterans do not negate the evidence from RCTs that the addition of SMBG and education can result in a decrease in A1c levels of about 0.3% absolute at six months and up to one year. As previously noted, I do not know why observational studies are included at all, and recommend that that the observational studies be removed.	Observational studies were included as the only available evidence of effectiveness in VA patients.
Pogach	Conclusions	The investigators, on multiple occasions state "that these studies do raise the question of whether veteran patients are receiving the full possible benefits of SMBG." It should be removed. Further, these statements indicate to me a pre-conceived bias, especially since the issue of SMBG efficacy, in individuals who are diet controlled or stable is controversial, and cannot be fully resolved by a meta-analysis. Furthermore, and this is more pertinent to the issue, the investigators indicated that "we draw no conclusion about the effect of frequency of SMBG monitoring on A1c values, and judge the strength of the evidence to be very low."	We disagree with the suggestion to remove the statement about effectiveness of SMBG in Veterans, as there is evidence to support no effectiveness.
Pogach	Future Research	One important limitation of the meta-analysis is that earlier studies from the early mid-90s used SMBG methodology that was much more inconvenient than current methodology. Glucose meters from that era required substantially more blood, transfer to the monitoring strip was more cumbersome, and data feedback from the meters less user friendly if present at all. All of these factors may have contributed to inconclusive results from early studies, and emphasizes the need for research in this area.	We have added this to future research
Pogach	Future Research	The investigators note: "The evidence is insufficient to draw conclusions about which components of SMBG (additional-education, algorithms or other techniques to adjust medication) and frequency of testing are most associated with better results. More research is needed." Agree, this limitation is important and should be better highlighted.	We added additional text on this.
Pogach	Future Research	"However, observational studies in the VA do not report differences in A1c levels between Veterans using or not using SMBG supplies. This raises the question about implementation: more research is needed to understand if implementation of SMBG in a typical VA clinic setting is sufficient for Veterans to receive the full benefit reported in clinical trials." The more pertinent issue is efficacy not effectiveness (see item 2). Please delete this statement.	We disagree, and note that VA's key question to us concerned effectiveness as well as efficacy.
Pogach	Future Research	"Additionally, data are needed about the cost-effectiveness of SMBG in a VA setting.". This seems premature to me. Even if such data were available, it would also involve a number of assumptions that would have to be based upon Markov modeling.	We agree this would involve modeling, but disagree that such an effort is premature. Our analysis of efficacy data support that SMBG is efficacious, therefore a CEA analysis may help better determine which variables are most important in determining cost effectiveness and the identification of these important variables could then target new studies.
Pogach	Future Research	Impact of SMBG on medication adherence should be evaluated. Non-compliance with oral-antiglycemic medications is a recognized issue among veterans and among non-veterans. It is also possible the system interventions to improve adherence may not need to incorporate increased frequency of SMBG.	We have added this to future research.
Pogach	Future Research	I have noted my comments about the Cho/Kwon study design in the previous section. Nonetheless, although I have some reservations about the study design for the purpose of this meta-analysis given the author's inclusion/exclusion criteria, I think that the study design is actually more relevant to what is now considered usual care; e.g., most persons with type 2 diabetes with training in SMBG and some supplies. (Key question 4). This might be mentioned under future research; i.e., that usual care (infrequent) for SMBG be the control group for persons with diabetes on oral agents.	We added this to future research.

Peer Review Comments Table 1. Continued

Reviewer	Section	Comment	Change
Aron	Future Research	This section seems pretty generic for the most part. More problematic is that SMBG is viewed completely in isolation. Most diabetes interventions are complex and involve more than activity. Moreover, other outcomes are relevant, e.g., behavior change. Finally, what does pramlintide have to do with this? That seemed to come out of the blue.	We have revised the future research section and also deleted the reference to pramlintide.
Pogach	Future Research	I substantially disagree with the language of the research implications. "Our review of existing data support the beneficial effect of SMBG on A1c levels in the context of a clinical trial. Although improvement in A1c is modest, it is equivalent to that achieved with some of the newer medical therapies for diabetes, such as pramlintide.44,45" As noted previously, I believe that there is a bias by including the Cho and Kwan studies. However, based upon the main analysis of this study, it is probably most pertinent to note that the benefit of SMBG [including bundled interventions] for persons on oral hypoglycemic agents is similar to that found for diabetes education interventions, many of which included SMBG (Norris et al, Diabetes Care, 2002). Better designed prospective clinical trials, especially for individuals with stable glycemic control (e.g., at their target A1c) are necessary. Mentioning a specific medication is inappropriate. Please delete.	We have dropped the use of pramlintide as a reference for efficacy and have inserted the diabetes education.
Pogach	Future Research	I would recommend, as noted previously, that future research include alternative study designs to reflect the fact that SMBG is considered usual care for patients on medication (though not on diet alone).	We made this change.
Pogach	Future Research	Use of SMBG in context of VHA Health Buddy would be an appropriate area of investigation.	We added this to future research.
Pogach	Overall Evaluation	The investigators were thorough in their identification of possible trials for inclusion in their report, but the reviewer has concerns that the included randomized trials articles from Cho and Kwan did not meet the stated inclusion criteria. This introduces biases which are not fully addressed in their discussion/and conclusions. This is a significant flaw of the study as written, and it needs to be more fully addressed. If the investigators wish to justify their inclusion, then the reviewer suggests that the meta-analysis should be presented with and without these studies to permit comparison with the AHRQ evidence synthesis.	We agree that leaving in Cho and Kwon introduced biased and have therefore removed them from the analyses in this revision.

APPENDIX C. EVIDENCE TABLE

Evidence Table 1. Randomized Controlled Trials Evaluating the Self-Monitoring of Blood Glucose

Author, Year	Sample Size Enroll/Follow-up	Dur. of Diabetes in Years	Mean Age	Mean Weight (kg)/BMI	% Women / Race	Allocation Concealment	Similarity at Baseline between groups	Outcome assessor blind	Care provider blind	Patients blinded	Did analysis included intention to treat analysis	Sample Size entering	Components	# Visit	Freq of SMBG Times/Week	Dur. of Tx	Outcome	Adverse Events
Wing RR et al., 1986 [19]	50 / 45	NR	54	98 / NR	78% / NR	Yes	Yes	Yes	No	No	Yes	25	Exercise; Counseling/Edu	20	Control	62 wks	A1c; Fasting Glucose; BMI/Weight loss	ND
									No	No		25	SMBG; Exercise; Pt Control led; Counseling/Edu	20	5.4	62 wks		
Fontbonne A et al., 1989 [20]	208 / 164	13	55	73 / 27	42% / NR	No	No	Yes	No	No	No	68	Counseling/Edu	4	Control	6 mths	A1c; BMI/Weight Loss	ND
						Yes		No	No	No		68	SMBG; Counseling/Edu	4	7.5	6 mths		
Rutten G et al., 1990 [23]	149 / 127	8.1	63	75 / NR	65% / NR	No	No	Yes	No	No	Yes	83	NR	NA	Control	1 year	A1c; BMI/Weight Loss	ND
						No		No	No	No		66	Counseling/Edu	Variable	NR	1 year		
Muchmore DB et al., 1994 [24]	29 / 23	5	59	99 / 34	61% / NR	Yes	Yes	Yes	No	No	Yes	14	Dietician; Counseling/Edu	8	Control	44 wks	A1c; BMI/Weight Loss; HRQOL*	ND
						No	Yes	No	No	No	Yes	15	SMBG; Dietician; Counseling/Edu	8	3	44 wks		
Jaber LA et al., 1996 [25]	45 / 39	6	62	90 / 33	70% / African Ancestry	No	No	Yes	No	No	Yes	22	NR	2	Control	4 mths	A1c; Fasting Glucose; HRQOL*	Hypoglycemia
						No		No	No	No	No	23	SMBG; Pt Controlled; Counseling/Edu	NR	8	4 mths		
Kibriya MG, et al., 1999 [27]	64 / 64	NR	50	60 / 24	45% / NR	No	No	Yes	No	No	Yes	32	Counseling/Edu	19	Control	18 mths	A1c; Fasting Glucose	Hypoglycemia
						No		No	No	No	No	32	SMBG; Pt Control led; Counseling/Edu	7	1	18 mths		
Schwedes U, et al., 2002 [29]	250 / 223	5.3	60	89 / 31	48% / NR	Yes	Yes	Yes	No	No	Yes	110+	Counseling/Edu	6	Control	24 wks	A1c; BMI/Weight Loss; HRQOL*	ND
						No	Yes	No	No	No	No	113+	SMBG; Dietician; Counseling/Edu	6	12	24 wks		
Guerci B, et al., 2003 [30]	988 / 689	8.1	62	83 / 30	45% / NR	No	No	Yes	No	No	Yes	344+	Counseling/Edu	5	Control	6 mths	A1c; Fasting Glucose	Hypoglycemia; Other
						No	Yes	No	No	No	Yes	345+	SMBG; Counseling/Edu	5	6	6 mths		
Davidson MB, et al., 2005 [31]	89 / 88	5.6	50	82.3 / 32.5	74% / African Ancestry, Hispanic, Other	No	No	Yes	No	No	Yes	45	Dietician; Other	13	Control	6 mths	A1c; BMI/Weight Loss	ND
						No	Yes	Yes	Yes	No	Yes	43	SMBG; Dietician; Other	13	36	6 mths		
Farmer A et al., 2007 [33]	453 / 453	3	66	NR / 31.3	43% / NR	Yes	Yes	Yes	No	No	Yes	152	Usual Care	NR	Control	12 mths	A1c; BMI/Weight Loss	Hypoglycemia
						Yes		No	No	No	Yes	150	SMBG	NR	6	12 mths		
						Yes		No	No	No	Yes	151	SMBG; Patient Control	NR	NR	12 mths		

ND=Not Described, NR=Not Reported, NA=Not applicable, *HRQOL=Health Related Quality of Life, +No entering sample size reported, this is the sample size completing the trial

www.ingramcontent.com/pod-product-compliance
Lightning Source LLC
Chambersburg PA
CBHW081623170526
45166CB00009B/3083